Everything You Need to Know About Relationship Violence

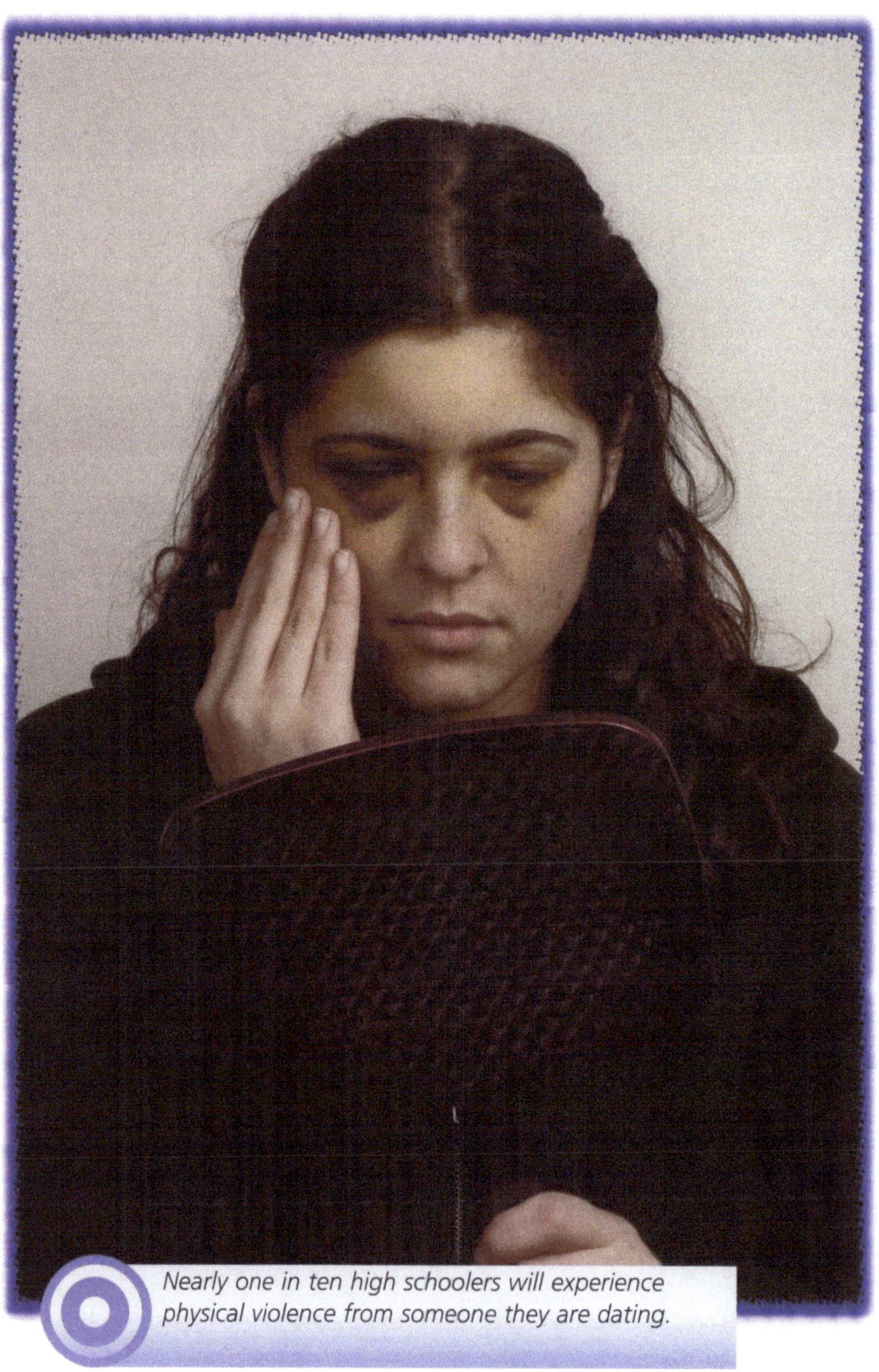

Nearly one in ten high schoolers will experience physical violence from someone they are dating.

Everything You Need to Know About Relationship Violence

Katherine White

The Rosen Publishing Group, Inc.
New York

Published in 2001 by The Rosen Publishing Group, Inc.
29 East 21st Street, New York, NY 10010

Copyright © 2001 by The Rosen Publishing Group, Inc.

First Edition

All rights reserved. No part of this book may be reproduced in any form without permission in writing from the publisher, except by a reviewer.

Library of Congress Cataloging-in-Publication Data

White, Katherine, 1975–
Everything you need to know about relationship violence / by Katherine White.— 1st ed.
p. cm. — (Need to know library)
Includes bibliographical references and index.
ISBN 978-1-4358-8737-4
1. Dating violence—Juvenile literature. 2. Interpersonal relations in adolescence—Juvenile literature. [1. Dating violence.] I. Title. II. Series.
HQ801.83 .W56 2001
306.73—dc21

00-012137

Manufactured in the United States of America

Contents

	Introduction	6
Chapter 1	The Truth About Dating Violence	10
Chapter 2	The Increase in Dating Violence	20
Chapter 3	What Is a Healthy Relationship?	30
Chapter 4	Moving On	39
	Glossary	54
	Where to Go for Help	56
	For Further Reading	60
	Index	62

Introduction

Relationships are one of the most important and intricate parts of your life. Whether it is the relationship you have with your parents, siblings, friends, or boyfriend or girlfriend, your relationships shape much of who you are and what you know about the world around you. They are supposed to teach you good things—how to communicate, love, compromise, and enjoy others. But some relationships do not do this. Instead, they hurt you, making you question yourself and all the things you have been taught to believe in. These are called abusive relationships, and teens are beginning to have to deal with them more and more, particularly with a specific type of abuse called dating violence.

Introduction

You would think that since abusive relationships, especially ones that involve violence, are bad for you, it would be easy to walk away from them. As you will learn in this book, however, abusive relationships are very hard to get out of, and sometimes even harder to recognize—especially for a teen whose abuser is his or her boyfriend or girlfriend.

In March 1998, at Columbia University in New York City, a young woman was slain by her boyfriend, resulting in him taking his own life only a few hours later. Unfortunately, this incident is not an isolated one. Just a few days after the Columbia University murder, a young man in Westchester County in New York State shot his girlfriend, critically wounding her, then killed himself right afterward.

Dating violence has been increasing fast. A recent survey found that 28 percent of high school and college students experience violence while dating. In fact, nearly one in ten high schoolers will experience physical violence with someone they are going out with. Sadly, falling in love is one of the reasons being a teenager is so fascinating, and also why this time in your life is so hard. Your first crush, date, and kiss will make you feel like you are soaring through life. Suddenly, it won't matter so much that your hair is sometimes frizzy or that your parents can be so overprotective, because the boy or girl whom you have

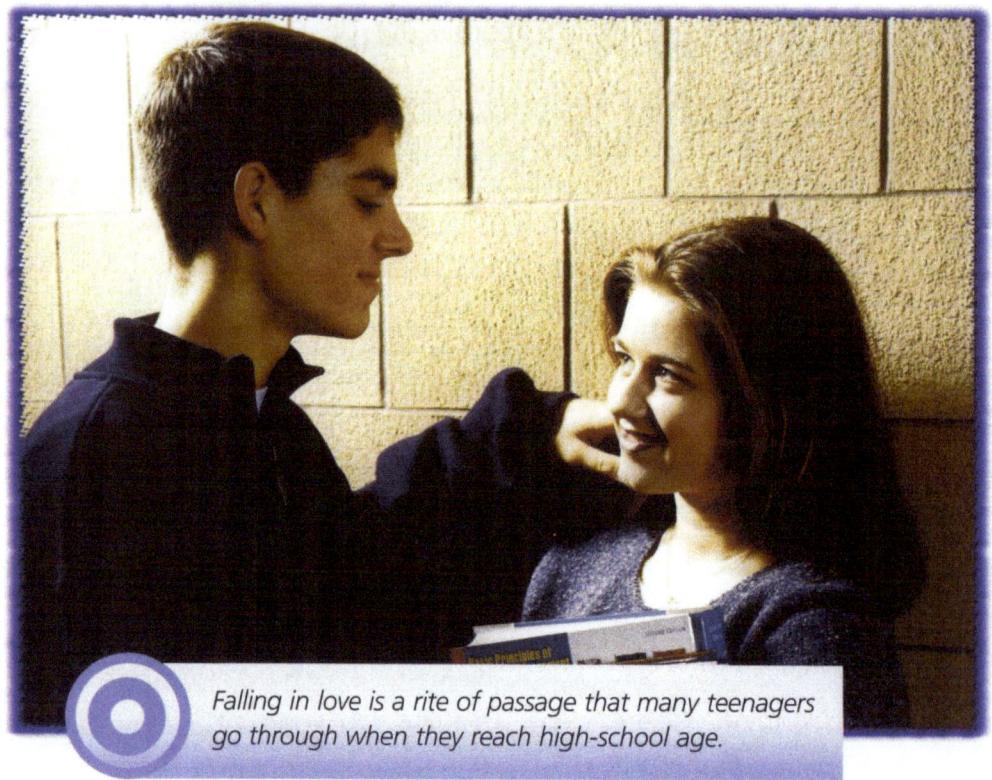

Falling in love is a rite of passage that many teenagers go through when they reach high-school age.

stared at for a whole year, hoping that he or she would notice you, finally has.

But how does that perfect feeling, that dream, turn into a raging nightmare? And how do you know when it has? What makes an argument, just that, an argument, and not a form of abuse? And if your relationship has become violent, how do you get out of it safely and move on with your life?

This book will answer each of these questions and more. It will explain the various types of abuse that can occur in a relationship, concentrating on violence. We will examine what makes a relationship healthy, as well as what to look for if you think you are in an unhealthy

Introduction

relationship, especially a violent one. We will also go deeper and explore the reasons why teens may be resorting to violence more often. We will shatter the myth that only men abuse women. Finally, we will talk about what to do if you or someone you know is in a violent relationship, and discuss how you can help yourself, or your friend, to end the suffering.

Remember, relationships are supposed to heighten your happiness, not drag you down. As a teenager, you have so much to deal with already; having a boyfriend or girlfriend is just not worth it if you begin fearing for your safety or even your life.

Chapter 1
The Truth About Dating Violence

Andrea and Miguel had been going out for three months. They hung out at lunch and after school, and then they talked on the phone every night. Miguel was so nice to Andrea. Whatever she wanted, he did it. Like if she said she wanted flowers, the next morning at school Miguel would be waiting at Andrea's locker with a bunch of tulips, her favorite. All of Andrea's friends were amazed at how well he treated her. "She's my princess," Miguel would tell anyone who would listen.

But Andrea was getting kind of tired of having to hang out with Miguel all the time. She missed her friends, but it wasn't a big deal

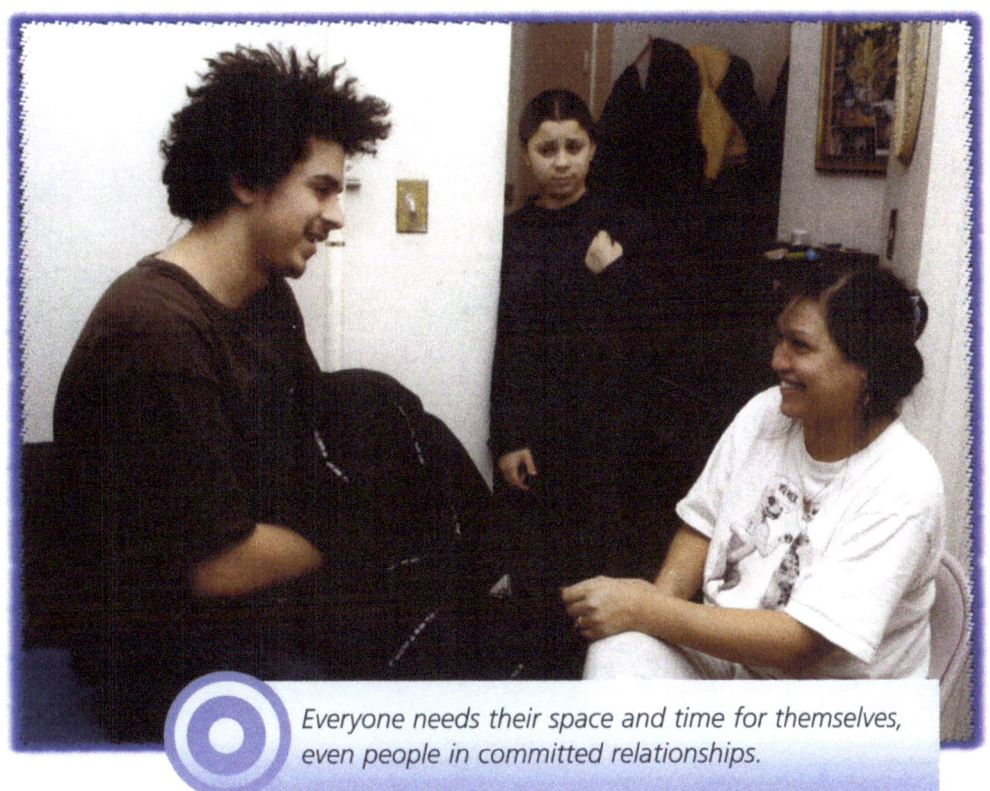

Everyone needs their space and time for themselves, even people in committed relationships.

because basketball had begun, so she had a reason not to be with him.

That's when it started. Andrea would get home from practice and Miguel would be waiting for her, hanging out with her parents. At first, it didn't seem weird. She just thought he missed her. But then after a week of getting home and Miguel being there, Andrea said something. "Miguel, some nights it would be cool if I could just come home and relax without you, you know. I need my privacy and time to do my homework."

"Are you breaking up with me? Is that what you want? Are you seeing someone else?"

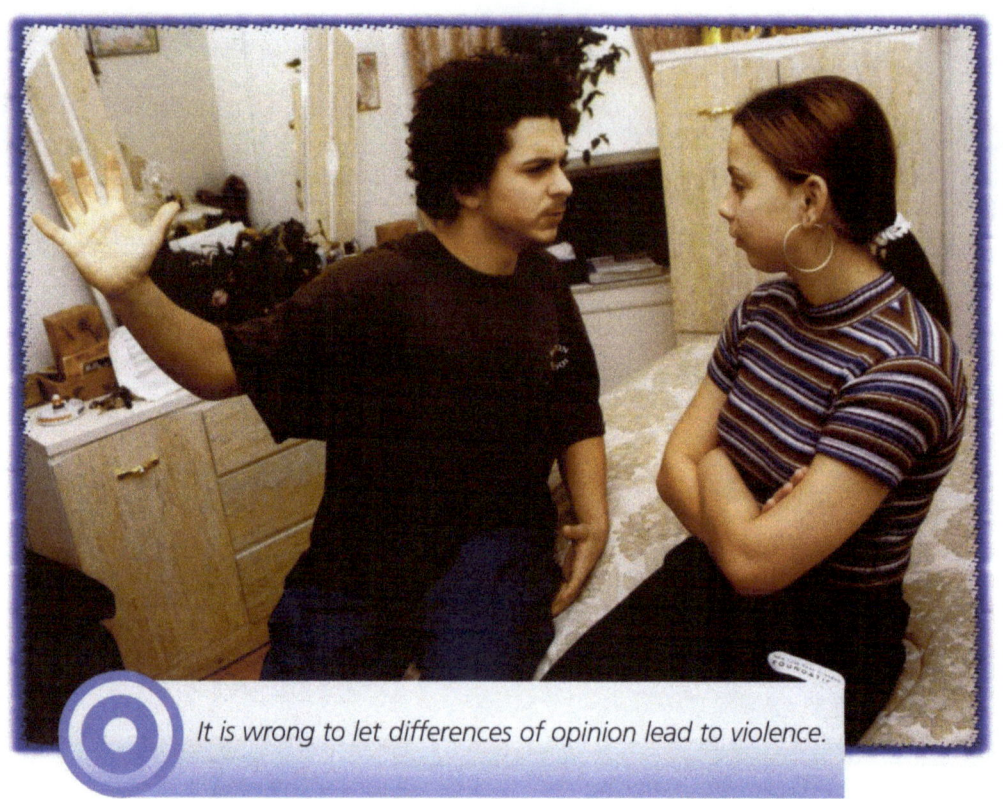

It is wrong to let differences of opinion lead to violence.

"No, Miguel. I just want some time for me, OK?"

"It's Andrew, isn't it? You don't want me around so he can come over. I knew you were cheating on me!"

"What are you talking about? I don't like Andrew. I like you."

"Whatever," Miguel said, as he walked toward Andrea. "I know you think you're better than me. I knew it all along. I'm so nice to you, why would you like anyone else ever, huh?"

"Miguel, you're freaking me out!"

"Shut up!" he screamed, as he slapped Andrea across her face.

The Truth About Dating Violence

What Is Dating Violence?

As Miguel slapping Andrea illustrates, dating violence is any intentional attack—physical or psychological—that is being done to you by your boyfriend or girlfriend. Andrea has become involved in dating violence and has a violent relationship to deal with. According to the Texas Council on Family Violence, the exact definition of dating violence is "a pattern of behavior used by an individual to maintain control over his or her dating partner."

Dating violence can disguise itself in many ways, meaning it doesn't have to be a slap or punch. Your partner could manipulate you into doing things you do not want to do or constantly tell you that you are stupid. It can be abrupt, for instance, if you're walking down the street and suddenly your girlfriend just explodes on you. However, a lot of times, dating violence happens when tensions are high, possibly during an argument or debate that gets out of control. But does that make it OK? Perhaps you just said something that really hurt your girlfriend, so it feels like she was not right, but not quite wrong in her response. Maybe she just didn't know what else to do.

Think about it: Even though it may have happened only once, the person you love has been abusive toward you. Also, considering that 70 percent of serious injuries and deaths occur when an abused

Relationship Violence

person is trying to leave or has already left a relationship, violent tendencies are a serious matter and you need to be exceptionally careful when dealing with a person who has them. Remember, though, dating violence is not only physical abuse. It can also be verbal/emotional or sexual abuse.

Physical Abuse

It is never OK for anyone to hit or slap you, whether it is your parent, friend, or boyfriend or girlfriend. No matter if he or she is having a rough day or is drinking and things just seem to get out of control, this is not a reason or an excuse. Violence should not happen, ever. This is why physical abuse is defined as any behavior that inflicts harm on a person. If someone shoves you, pulls your hair, bites you, or even throws an object at you, he or she is physically abusing you.

Verbal Abuse/Emotional Abuse

Karen and Peter had been together for six months when Karen started thinking all these strange things. When she and Peter weren't together, she would imagine him looking at other girls and flirting with them. Karen knew that Peter was a great boyfriend, but she couldn't shake the feeling that he wasn't in love with her. So why wouldn't he be flirting with other girls?

The Truth About Dating Violence

Although Karen never told Peter what she was thinking, he picked up on her change in behavior. So he sat her down and told her what he thought. "Karen, it's like we can't be apart. You get angry when I hang out with my friends, and you never want to hang out with yours anymore. You yell at me if I make a decision you don't like, and you cry all the time."

"So what, Peter!" Karen screamed. "We should want to spend time together. You always have so much to do, and you don't make me feel good about myself. Sometimes, I hate you. You're not even nice. I think you're probably the worst boyfriend anyone has ever had!"

"Karen, you always say things like that to me. Why are you with me then?"

Obviously, Karen and Peter are having some problems, and not only with communication. Karen's lack of trust is causing her to verbally abuse Peter. Verbal abuse is behavior that causes harm with words. If someone calls you names, criticizes you, ignores you, humiliates you, or yells at you, you are being verbally assaulted. Often, verbal abuse is hard to recognize because it doesn't leave physical marks. You're not bruised or battered, but it quickly lowers your self-esteem and makes you feel worthless.

Relationship Violence

Dating Violence in Same-Sex Relationships

The Columbia/Barnard Rape Crisis/Anti-Violence Support Center reports that "relationship violence happens in same-sex relationships at about the same rate as in heterosexual relationships." It is incredibly hard for any teen to tell someone they are being abused, and homosexual teens have an added burden. Many times, if they are being abused, they stay quiet because if they do tell someone, the chances that they will be forced to "come out" are greatly increased. If a teen is not ready for this step, he or she often remains silent about the abuse out of fear that his or her sexuality will be discovered.

Emotional abuse is born out of verbal abuse. It is any behavior intended to cause psychological or emotional distress. This can be in the form of threats, put-downs, jealousy, possessiveness, or isolating someone from his or her friends or family. Karen was also emotionally abusing Peter because she was jealous and didn't want to ever let him out of her sight. She thought that by controlling him, he would not get the opportunity to flirt with other girls.

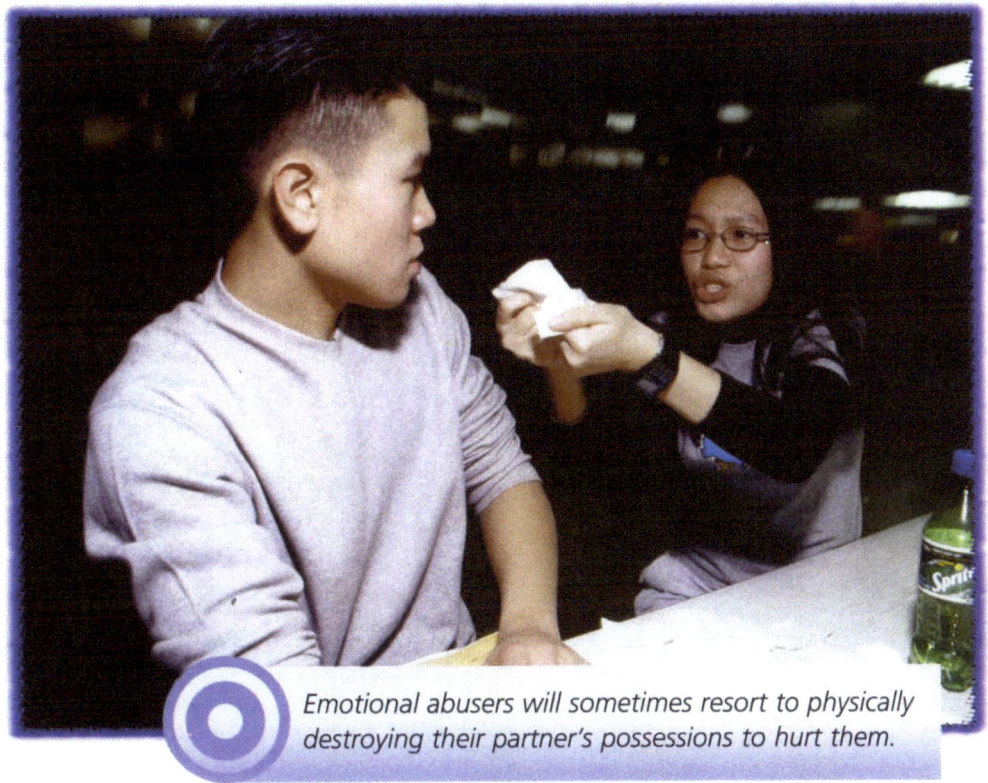

Emotional abusers will sometimes resort to physically destroying their partner's possessions to hurt them.

In extreme forms of emotional abuse, the abuser may even resort to destroying gifts, clothes, or letters, or damaging his or her partner's most prized possessions.

Sexual Abuse

Sexual abuse is sex that is forced or any sexual behavior that makes a person feel uncomfortable. It can range from your brother's friend making sexual comments about you, to your boyfriend or girlfriend manipulating you to have sex. Lines like "If you loved me, you would . . . " or "Everybody else does it" are definitely forms of sexual abuse.

Relationship Violence

Relationship Violence Test

- Does my date ever hit, slap, shove, kick, or restrain me?
- Does my date ever threaten to hurt me?
- Does my date call me names or insult me?
- Does my date become jealous if I talk to or go places with other people?
- Does my date make me tell him or her where I am all the time?
- Does my date blame alcohol or drugs for becoming angry or losing control?
- Does my date ever touch me without my permission or force me to have sex against my will?
- Does my date threaten to commit suicide if I try to leave the relationship?
- Am I afraid to disagree with my date?
- When I spend time with other people, does my date become angry and accuse me of cheating?
- Do I avoid seeing friends or doing things because I'm afraid my date will get angry?

The Truth About Dating Violence

What to Do If You're Not Sure

Although dating violence seems easy to recognize, it is often a struggle for teens to identify it as a problem when it happens in a real-life relationship. This is why the Adolescent Health Initiative of the West Virginia Bureau for Public Health has come up with a test that will help you know if you are involved in dating violence. If you can answer yes to any of the questions on the facing page, you are involved in a violent relationship. If you realize that your relationship is a violent one, please contact one of the sources that are listed in the Where to Go for Help section in the back of this book.

It is upsetting to think that while you are dating you have to be alert for signs of dating violence, especially because, as a teenager, it is very normal to want a fairy-tale relationship—one that is perfect, free of problems, and straight-up fiction. In reality, relationships are a tangle of experiences, past to present. Even psychologists struggle to identify what causes a relationship to turn violent. Is it just that two people's personalities do not mesh, or is it the high profile of violence in our society—on television, in movies, and in video games? Could it stem from a teen coming from an abusive home and experiencing violence from the time he or she was a child? The next chapter will talk about these issues and discuss the reasons why dating violence happens.

Chapter 2: The Increase in Dating Violence

As reported by Callie Marie Rennison, Ph.D., and Sarah Welchans in their book *Intimate Partner Violence*, "Women experienced the highest rates of intimate partner violence between 1993 and 1998." Reporting a similar pattern, the Corporate Alliance to End Partner Violence reports that "one in five college students report at least one incident of abuse when dating." These statistics tell a scary tale. Dating violence is becoming a very big problem. Psychologists and sociologists are now studying the reasons dating violence is happening more and more.

Reasons for Violence

The fact that more teens are beginning to be overwhelmed with adult issues, like pregnancy and drinking, at a younger age causes a lot of stress during a

The Increase in Dating Violence

stage of life that is already incredibly confusing. Add in the extreme violence that is shown on television and in movies, and the fact that parents and teens are becoming more isolated from one another, and the increase in dating violence becomes a bit clearer. Violent behavior is being presented in popular culture, yet not being discussed at home, and so teens may start releasing their frustrations through violence.

Media Violence

It is a major concern that violence in the media is contributing to the increase in violent behavior among teens. Video games, television shows, and movies show brutal fight scenes and arguments that look completely real. In fact, as violent scenes become more realistic, many researchers are studying whether teens are learning their violent responses from these shows or games.

Teens are also spending more time than ever before watching these shows and movies and playing these games. For example, rather than hanging out with their friends, teens are choosing to stay inside to watch television and surf the Internet, another place excessive violence can be found.

The Vicious Circle

It had been happening for years, and Kristina had known it was wrong every single time it happened. She would sit in her room as her parents argued, and she could hear when the hitting

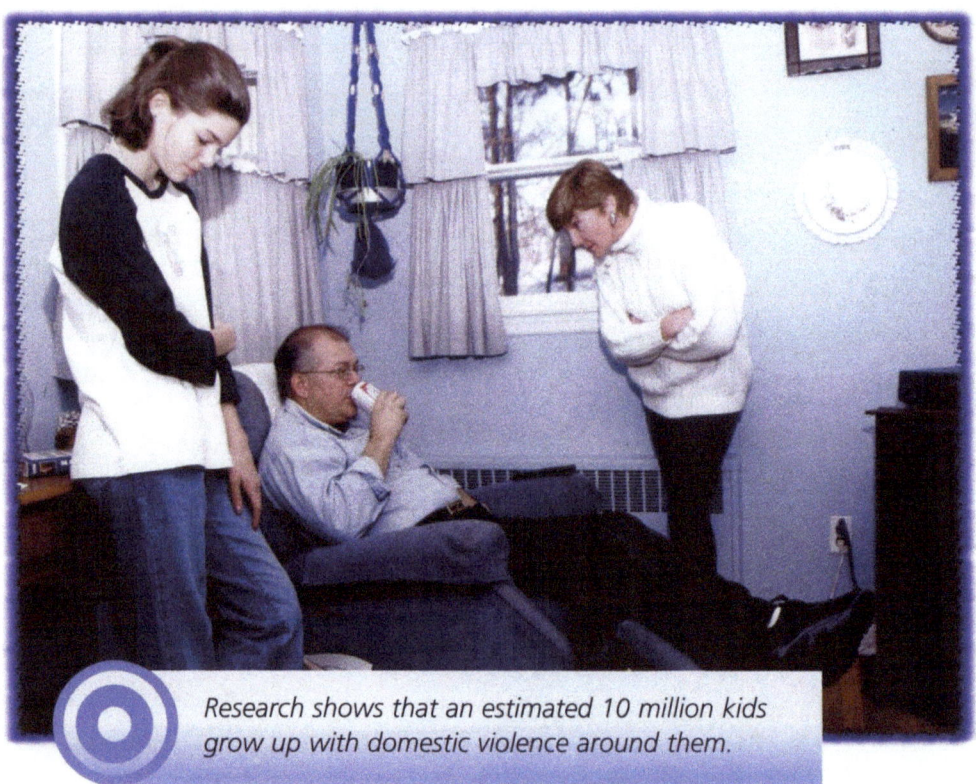

Research shows that an estimated 10 million kids grow up with domestic violence around them.

started. Her mom would be screaming at her dad for drinking too much, telling him that he was neglecting his family, and her dad would just ignore her as he sat watching television.

This would go on for at least fifteen minutes until her mom would get so angry she would start throwing things at Kristina's dad. It was horrible. Anything she could find she would throw at him. And then came the violence.

Her dad would stand up and scream at her mom to stop it, and her mom would yell every obscenity she could think of. Then they would start hitting each other and chasing each other

The Increase in Dating Violence

through the house. The next morning, though, when Kristina got up, everything would seem normal again.

Since Kristina knew it was wrong, she just ignored them, never thinking they were affecting her. But when she was a senior in high school, she started dating a great guy named Adam. The first six months were beautiful; they never fought once. But one night, Adam and Kristina were at a party and Adam got really drunk. Kristina told him she wanted to leave and as she was driving them home, she started telling him how stupid he was to be drinking. Adam ignored her. That's when it hit.

Kristina started going crazy, screaming and yelling as loud as she could. She started driving really fast while she tried to hit Adam. When they came to a red light, Adam got out of the car. Kristina drove beside him up the street, yelling what a loser he was.

As more research is developed, it is becoming clear that a child who grows up in a violent home does not walk away untouched. Unfortunately, about 10 million kids grow up in such homes. In a recent study, it was found that the effects of being abused greatly increase a teen's chance of getting into an abusive relationship. In fact, 57 percent of adolescents who were abused as they were growing up find themselves becoming as abusive as their parents.

When children grow up in an abusive household, they do not learn how to deal with their anger. Instead, they gain a very warped perception of the role of men and women in the family. These perceptions are then carried into the child's teen years and into his or her adult life. When dating, all of these issues begin to surface because he or she has never learned how to develop a healthy relationship. Without the ability to cope with anger—and with the memories of how the parents coped—a teen who was raised in an abusive household tends to slip into old patterns.

Project PAVE (Providing Alternatives to Violence) is an organization that was created in response to this problem. Started in 1985, Project PAVE has counseled teens to teach them that violence is not the answer, even though it is the only answer they have ever learned. If you or someone you know would benefit from this organization, please see the Where to Go for Help section in the back of this book.

Drugs and Alcohol

During high school, and then again in college, many teens find themselves in social situations where alcohol or drugs are available. Saying no is the best possible answer for you and for your partner. Dating violence tends to happen more often when drugs and alcohol are

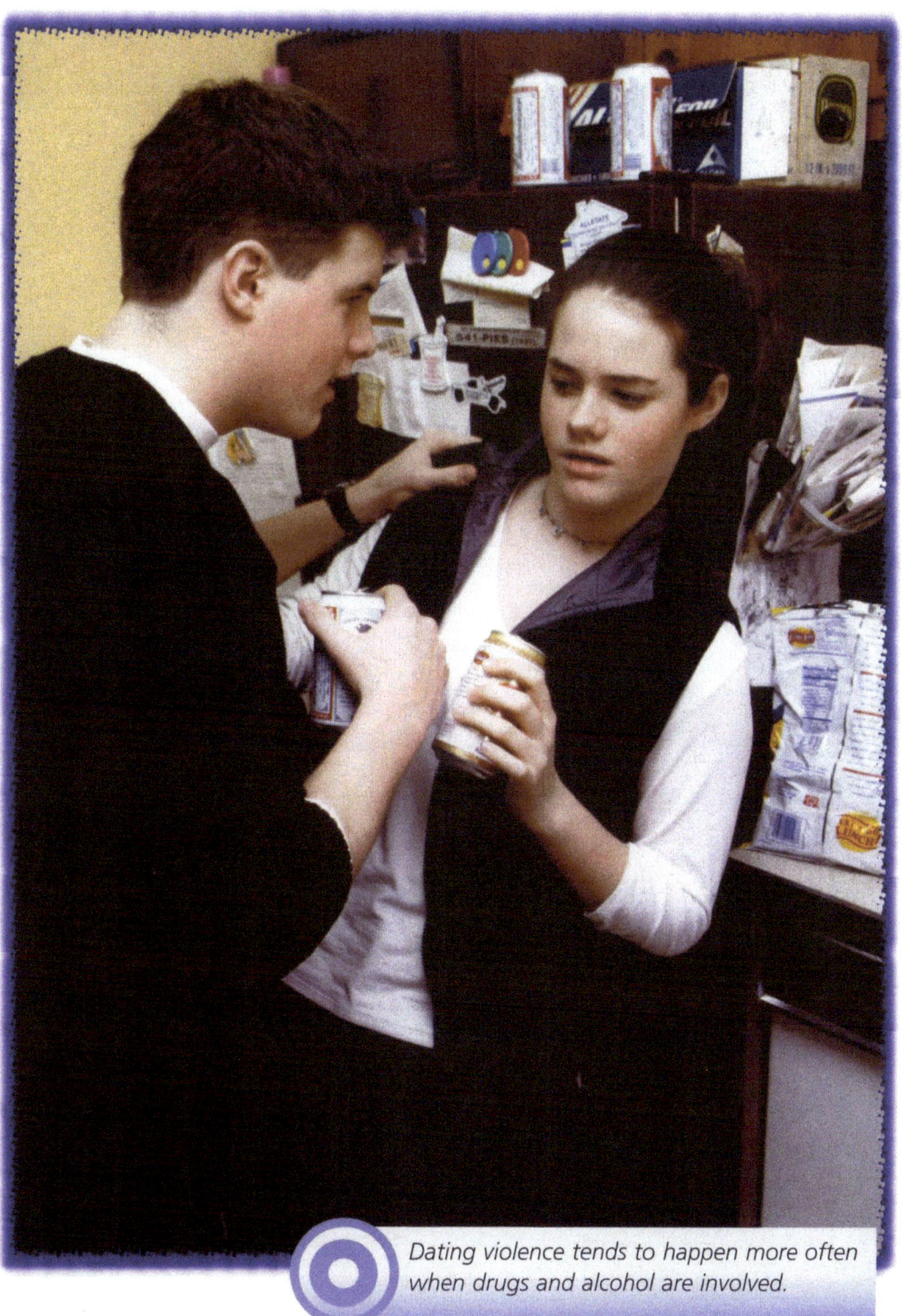
Dating violence tends to happen more often when drugs and alcohol are involved.

Relationship Violence

Myth: Women Are Not Abusers

Statistics show that although it is much more common for men to abuse women, women can and do abuse men, and it is on the rise. Most of the time, women do not respond with physical violence, which is why statistics make it seem like it does not occur. Instead, women use different forms of abuse, such as verbal or emotional, which also cause severe damage to a person and a relationship. Overall, abuse can be physical or mental. Marks do not have to be left on the skin for someone to be abused.

involved. Emotions run higher and self-control is lower, so the stage is set for violence.

However, it is important to recognize that alcohol is not an excuse for violent behavior, although many times abusers will use it as such. Aggressive tendencies are set in people's behavioral responses, not in the beer or hard liquor that they may have drunk. Instead, the alcohol has enhanced, or heightened, their inability to control their actions, so they end up turning their anger against those closest to them.

The Increase in Dating Violence

Teen Pregnancy

One of the most horrifying statistics about dating violence concerns teen mothers—over 70 percent of them are beaten by their boyfriends. And according to the National Campaign to Prevent Teen Pregnancy, "Four in ten young women become pregnant at least once before they reach the age of twenty—one million a year."

Being a mother, no matter how old you are, increases a lot of pressures. Women of all ages battle times of depression and a feeling of isolation from their husbands or boyfriends when they are pregnant. Teen mothers' responses tend to be even more intense, leaving them feeling very vulnerable and lacking in self-respect and self-esteem. They are often uncertain as to what is happening to their bodies and nervous about what they will confront in the future. And on top of all of this, they are trying to maintain relationships with their boyfriends. Again, tensions are high and, as can be seen from this startling statistic, the chance of violence is immense.

It should be obvious so far that it is never OK for your date to hurt you. But what might not be so obvious is what makes a relationship a good one. In the following chapter we will discuss what makes a relationship healthy and why, giving you the ability to compare healthy versus nonhealthy relationships. A

Relationship Violence

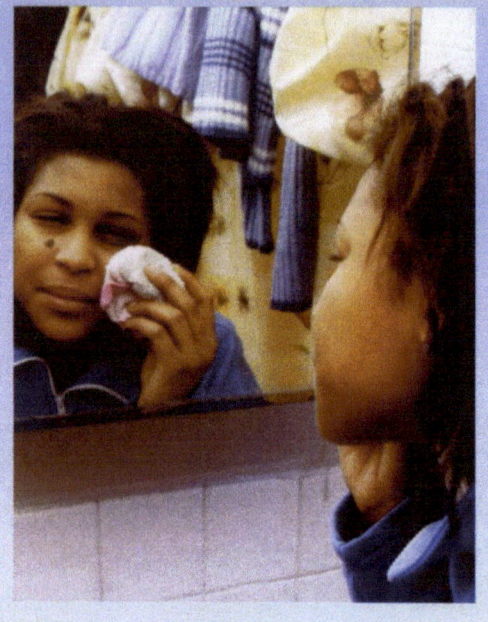

Violence Around the World

The United States is not the only country that has a problem with dating violence and abusive relationships. In a study done by the Johns Hopkins School of Public Health and Center for Health and Gender Equity, it was found that "around the world, one in three women has been beaten, coerced into sex, or otherwise abused during her lifetime."

In Japan, for example, the forms of abuse tend to be more than just physical, as they spread out into a range of psychological and sexual abuses as well. In a study that focused on Mexico, 52 percent of physically abused women had also been sexually abused by their partners. Facts like these show that changes need to come, and the world needs to start working toward them.

The Increase in Dating Violence

lot of times, it is easier to know when something is wrong if you first know what makes something right. Again, though, when talking about the positive characteristics of a relationship, we will also have to discuss the negative. For instance, if people know what makes a relationship healthy, why do they stay in ones that are not? Hopefully, by confronting these issues you will be able to not only recognize a healthy relationship, but know if you need to get out of an unhealthy one.

Chapter 3
What Is a Healthy Relationship?

Healthy relationships are something that everyone is seeking. No one wants to be in an unhealthy one, but the problem is, do you actually know what makes a relationship healthy? Is it healthy when your boyfriend or girlfriend does everything you ask? Is it healthy to spend all your time together? Is it OK to argue? When you think about dating this way, the definition of a healthy relationship may not seem so clear.

Respect

One of the most basic and fundamental aspects of a healthy relationship is respect. This ranges from respecting your partner's body to valuing his or her opinion. Something as simple as showing up on time when you plan to meet, or calling to let him or her know you are running late, is vital to being respectful. On the

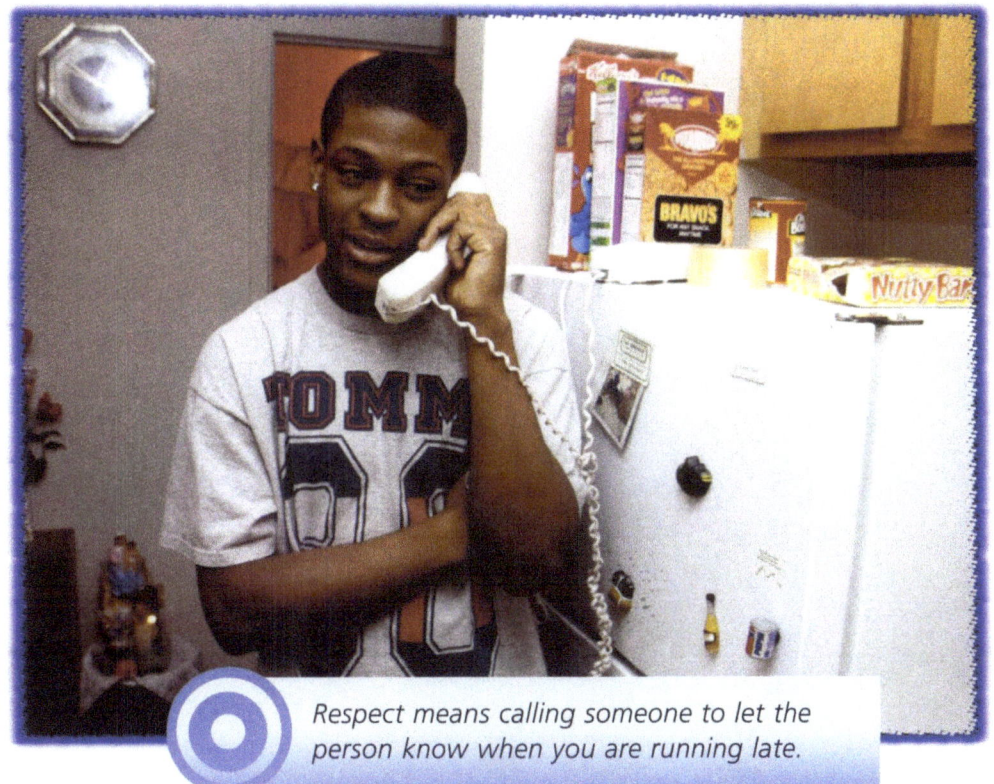
Respect means calling someone to let the person know when you are running late.

other hand, one of the trickier parts of respect is learning to understand and appreciate the differences between you and the person you are with, because there will be times when there is just no way you are going to see eye-to-eye. Acknowledging that your partner's idea is not necessarily wrong is a tough thing to do, especially if the discussion is about something you believe in. This is when communication becomes important.

Communication

In every relationship you have, you will eventually disagree about something. For example, your parents

Relationship Violence

might want you home at eleven when you want to come home at twelve, or your boyfriend could tell you that he can't go to the prom because he has to work. In both situations, expressing your ideas and feelings in the most articulate, or clearest, way possible is incredibly important. Screaming at your parents that everyone else gets to stay out late does not show them that you are able to communicate; neither does simply telling your boyfriend that you think he is a loser. Instead, explain why it is so important that you get that extra hour or tell your boyfriend why it would mean so much if he could get off work for the prom.

Communication is hard because sometimes, like in the case of the boyfriend working the night of the prom, you really can't understand why he doesn't know how important this night is to you. But maybe he really doesn't, or maybe he needs the money. This is why the second part of communication is listening.

Listen Up

Once you have explained, as honestly and openly as you can, why a particular belief or decision is important to you, it is time for you to be quiet and listen to the other person's side. While you are listening, try your best to look at your partner's side objectively, meaning without involving your personal feelings about the subject. This allows you to hear your partner's opinion with an open mind, and you will be more

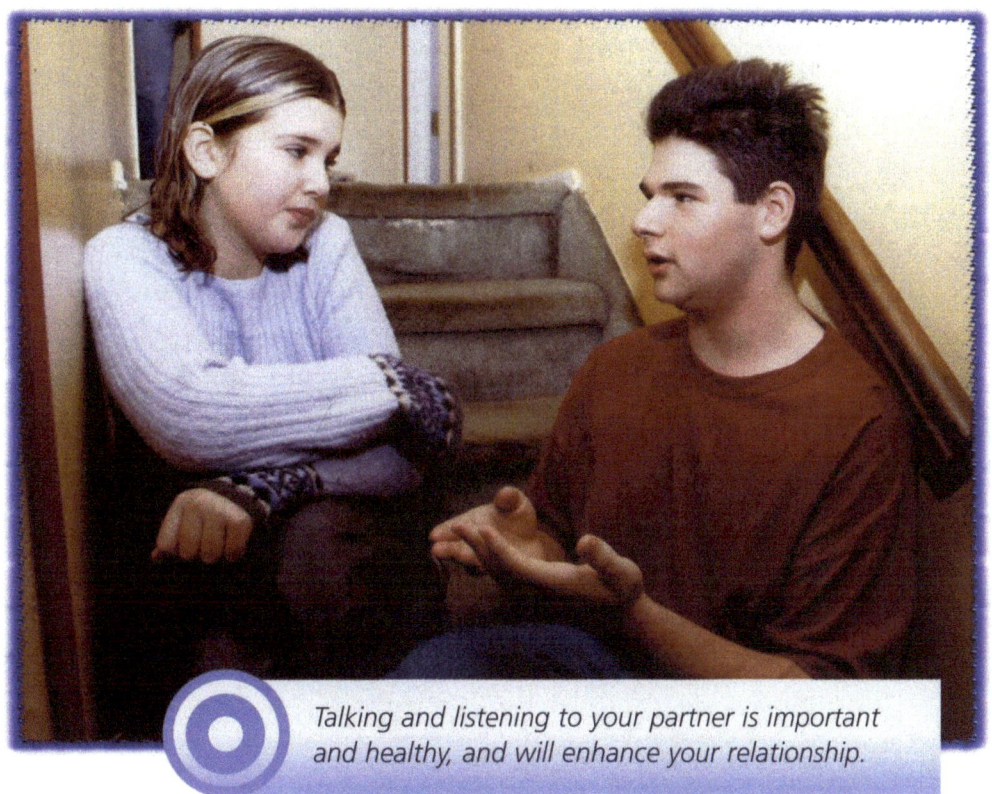

Talking and listening to your partner is important and healthy, and will enhance your relationship.

apt to understand exactly where they are coming from. If, for example, your boyfriend says that his dad is making him work the night of the prom, see if he will talk to his dad about it. But if he has to work for a good reason—not just because he doesn't want to go to the prom—then it is time to compromise.

Compromise

Once you and your boyfriend or girlfriend have explained your sides, what happens if you still can't agree? Compromise is an intricate process because, as you probably know, some people tend to be stubborn,

Relationship Violence

From the Los Angeles Commission on Assaults Against Women (LACAAW)

Bill of Rights for a Healthy Relationship

- I have the right to be treated with respect.
- I have the right to say no and not feel guilty.
- I have the right to change my mind.
- I deserve not to be hit.
- My partner deserves not to be yelled or screamed at.
- I do not deserve to be told that I'm stupid.
- I do not have the right to demand that my partner dress or act a certain way.

meaning they have a hard time seeing the other person's side. When you compromise, both sides have to give a little, meaning both people get a bit less than what they originally wanted. For example, in the previous case, the boyfriend could work for half of his shift and then come to the prom. A compromise has been reached.

What Is a Healthy Relationship?

Trust

Trust is also one of the most important factors in a relationship. Trust is believing that your partner is telling you the truth, and not being jealous and possessive. If your girlfriend tells you she is going out with her friends on Saturday night, and you trust her, you won't start imagining that she is really using this time to flirt with other guys. Many times, if people do not trust their partners, they will try to restrict their partner's activities or tag along. This is a form of control that stems from a lack of trust.

With the four key ingredients—respect, communication, compromise, and trust—a relationship can stay healthy and thrive. There are other important factors, like self-respect, that also play a part. If you can recognize these healthy tendencies in your relationship, you're on the right track. Keep in mind, though, that even if your relationship is based on these factors, unhealthy situations and patterns can arise.

Why Do People Stay?

It is often hard to leave a violent relationship. If you have never been in this type of situation, you may think, It just doesn't make sense—why would I stay if someone is hurting me? You're right, it doesn't make sense, although many teens can't see that at the time.

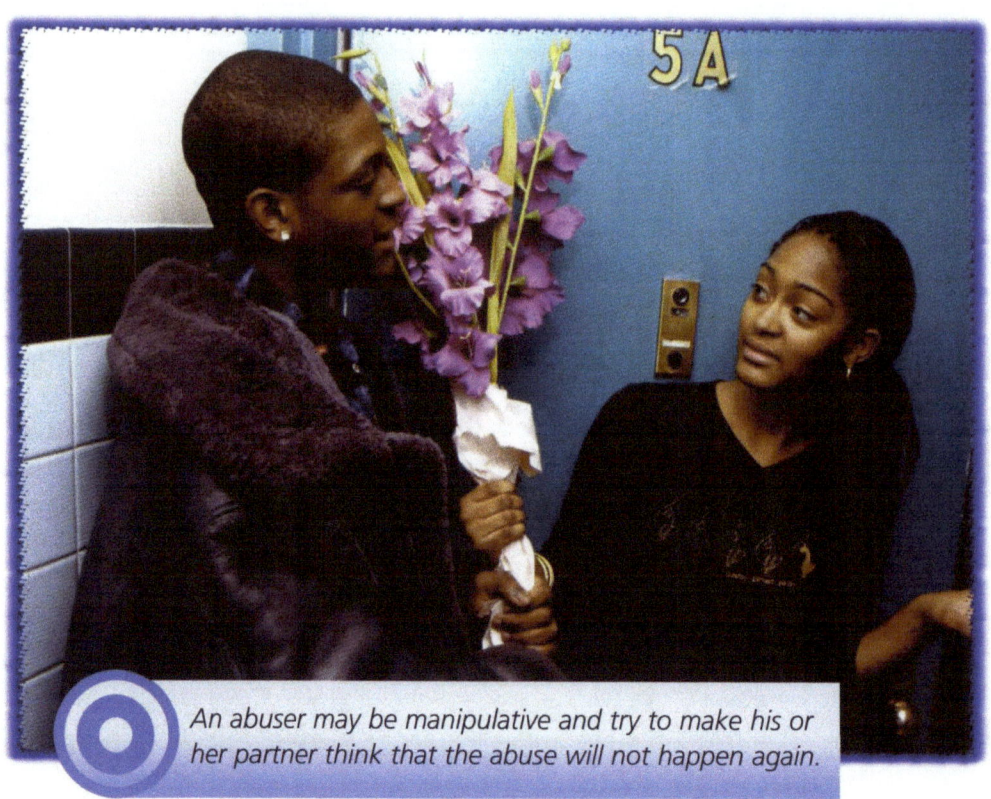

An abuser may be manipulative and try to make his or her partner think that the abuse will not happen again.

Excuses and Reasoning from the Abuser

One of the biggest reasons a person stays in a violent dating relationship is that the abuser often comes back and promises that it will never happen again. Often, he or she will express so much remorse that the partner may actually be manipulated into believing it was a mistake, a one-time thing. He or she may cry, bring flowers, and be exceptionally attentive, setting out to prove that this type of behavior is the exact opposite of who he or she is. And since the partner is in love, after a time, he or she accepts the apology, hoping that this is, indeed, the last time.

What Is a Healthy Relationship?

Healthy Vs. Unhealthy Behavior

Healthy Behavior

- Respecting your date and his or her friends and activities
- Keeping an open mind about your partner's beliefs and feelings
- Talking about your differences and opinions
- Communicating your feelings
- Both of you having an equal say in the relationship
- Finding solutions that work for both of you

Unhealthy Behavior

- Screaming and yelling at your date when you are angry
- Any form of violence
- Pouting to get what you want
- Believing that you have more rights and needs than your date

Relationship Violence

Excuses in the Mind of the Abused

No one wants to actually believe that they are in a violent relationship, so many times it is hard to admit when you are. It is difficult to accept that the person you fell in love with or are dating has a problem, especially when he or she is insistent that there is no problem, that it was just a horrible mistake. Too often, those who are being abused justify the violence in their minds, blaming it on stress, on the fact that their partners are going through a really hard time, or on themselves. For this reason, it is important to remember that there is no justification for violence. For example, it can't matter, even if it feels like it should, that your partner is stressed out or in pain because his or her parents recently got a divorce. You have to think about yourself and what is good and safe for you.

Now that you can recognize what makes a relationship healthy and what causes a person to stay in an abusive relationship, what happens if you decide you want to leave a violent relationship? How do you remove yourself from this dangerous situation in the safest way possible? The following chapter will talk about how you can safely leave an abusive relationship. It will also discuss how you can approach a friend who is in an abusive relationship, as well as some of the activities you can do to stop dating violence in your peer group and community.

Chapter 4: Moving On

Once you have recognized that you or someone you know is in an unhealthy or violent relationship, the next step is, obviously, to end it. However, just knowing that you or your friend needs to leave is only the first step. In fact, there are a few things you should do before you remove yourself or tell your friend to remove himself or herself from this dangerous situation.

If You Are Being Abused

If you are being abused, the first thing that you need to do is tell someone. This cannot be stressed enough. You may be in danger. Your life could be at stake. Your decision to leave needs to be shared with someone you can trust.

Relationship Violence

Telling Someone

The reason that talking with someone is so important is that you will need a lot of support in the coming days and months. Leaving an abusive relationship takes an enormous amount of strength, and often, by the time a person chooses to leave, his or her strength begins to fade. Telling someone what has been happening to you does not show that you are too weak to leave on your own. It shows that you are smart enough to recognize that leaving is going to be hard. But who should you talk to?

A Parent

Telling a parent or both of your parents what is going on in your life is a very good idea. They will then know not to take calls from the person who is harming you, or to let him or her anywhere near your home. This may sound strange, considering that you are a teenager and the last thing you want to admit is that you need your parents' help, but your parents can offer you protection. And right now, protection is what you need.

A Friend

If you know for certain that telling your parents is not a good idea, or if you just cannot bring yourself to let them in on what is happening, then you need to at least

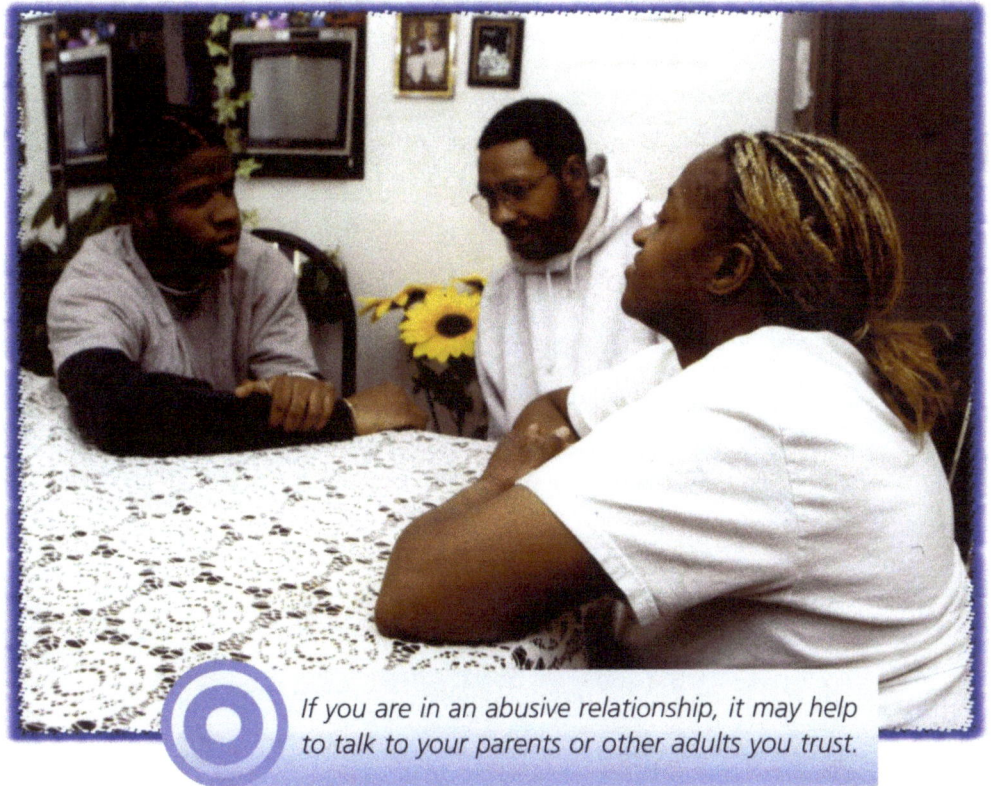
If you are in an abusive relationship, it may help to talk to your parents or other adults you trust.

tell a friend. Talking with a friend about your fears and concerns, as well as possible ways of leaving the relationship, will help you make sound decisions about how to proceed with your life.

However, keep in mind that telling a friend is not enough. You need to make an adult aware of the abuse. Perhaps you know a teacher, a friend's parent, or a counselor in school who you feel comfortable opening up to. No matter what, though, you do need to tell an adult because he or she will be able to help you cope with what is going on, and he or she can help you seek out other resources that can give you the support you need.

Relationship Violence

Intuition

When you are involved in dating violence, intuition is an ability that you must rely upon. Intuition is knowing that something is not right, without concrete evidence. A lot of times, when someone is involved in a violent relationship, they know intuitively that it is wrong. Deep down inside, even though they may cover it up, a person's intuition is screaming that this is not right! Yet by staying, hoping that the last hit was the last, he or she is not listening to himself or herself, and is definitely not following intuition.

If you are involved in a situation and it feels wrong—perhaps you do not know why exactly—remove yourself from it because it is wrong for you. If you listen to your own judgment, whether intuitive or concrete, you will decrease your chance of becoming caught in an abusive relationship.

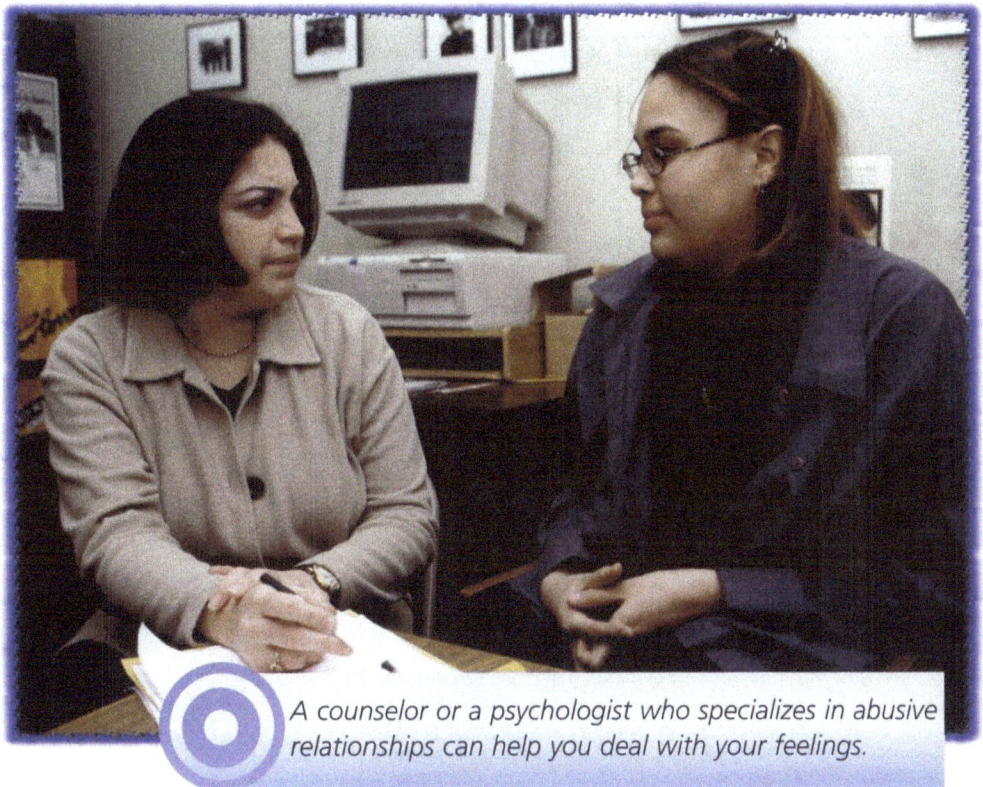

A counselor or a psychologist who specializes in abusive relationships can help you deal with your feelings.

Seeing a Counselor or Psychologist

If you are coming out of a violent or abusive relationship, it is a fact that you have just been through a very rough time. Ever heard the phrase "emotional roller coaster?" Well, you've just been riding one, and you may need a little help dealing with all the effects.

Earlier in the book, we talked about how abuse can lower your self-esteem, demolish your self-respect, and make you feel worthless as a person. This is very normal in this type of situation, and it is OK if you feel as though the things that are going through your mind are a bit overwhelming. A counselor or psychologist who

Relationship Violence

specializes in helping people who have been abused can help you sort through the upsetting feelings that you are left to deal with. They can also counsel you on the healthiest and safest way to leave the relationship so you can move on with your life. Most important, they can show you that the violence was not your fault.

Again, talking with someone is very important, and you should not think going to see a counselor or psychologist means you are crazy or insane. It does not. All it shows is that you realize that the time you have just gone through has been an incredibly hard one, and you are struggling to come to terms with it.

Staying Safe

Your biggest concern right now should be staying safe. The list below, from the LACAAW's relationship violence prevention curriculum, *In Touch with Teens*, gives you some guidelines on how you can do this. However, these guidelines should not take the place of talking to someone about the abuse.

General Safety

- **Stay in touch with your friends, and make it a point to spend time with people other than your partner.**

Moving On

- Stay involved in activities that you enjoy. Do not stop doing things that make you feel good about yourself.
- Take a self-defense class.
- Consider looking into resources at your school and in your community.
- Think about joining a support group or calling a crisis hotline.

Safety When Breaking Up with Your Partner

- Break up with your partner in a public place where other people are around.
- Tell other people that you plan to break up with your partner and tell them where you will be.
- Arrange to call a friend or a counselor after you talk with your partner so that you can talk about what happened.

Safety at School

- Always keep change with you so you can make phone calls.

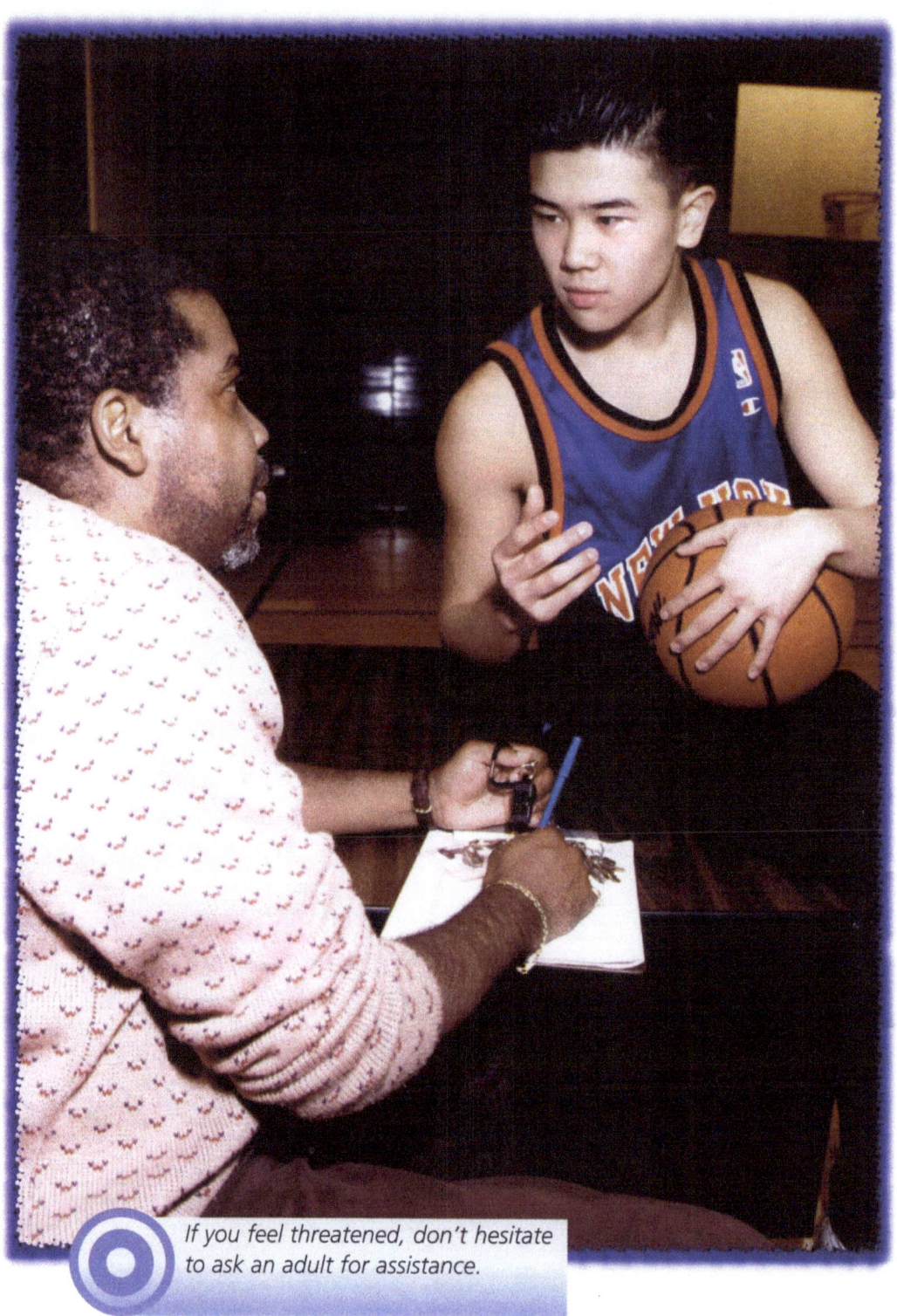

If you feel threatened, don't hesitate to ask an adult for assistance.

Moving On

- Try not to be alone.
- Tell teachers, counselors, coaches, or security guards about what is happening. Have them help you be safe.
- Change your routine. Don't always come to school the same way or arrive at the same time.
- Consider rearranging your class schedule.

Safety at Home

- Try not to be alone at home.
- Consider telling your parents or other family members about what is happening.
- Make a list of phone numbers. Included on this list should be emergency numbers like 911, as well as supportive friends you can call when you are upset.
- If you are home alone, make sure the doors are locked and windows are secure.

If Your Friend Is Being Abused

One of the hardest positions to be in as a friend is knowing or thinking that a friend of yours is in a violent or abusive relationship. Maybe you are not sure

Relationship Violence

what's the matter with your friend. You just know that his or her behavior has changed a lot over the past couple of months. Or maybe you don't think there is anything you can do. But, there is actually a lot you can do.

Symptoms of Violence

Recognizing that your friend is in an abusive relationship may not be easy—he or she may not tell you about it. You may just have a hunch about what is going on.

One of the biggest signs that someone is involved in a violent relationship is the presence of bruises, scrapes, or welts on his or her body. If you ask your friend what caused these injuries and he or she gives vague, or unclear, answers, you may have cause for concern. Another sign is a dramatic change in behavior. For instance, if your friend used to be outgoing and enjoy being with people but, since he or she got into this relationship, has been acting withdrawn and depressed, as well as reluctant to talk about why, you should be concerned.

Finally, how does your friend's partner treat him or her? Does the partner try to control your friend's every move or be with your friend all the time? Do you see them arguing a lot? Does the partner get really out of control? If you can answer yes to a few of these questions, you should at least talk to your friend about what you have noticed.

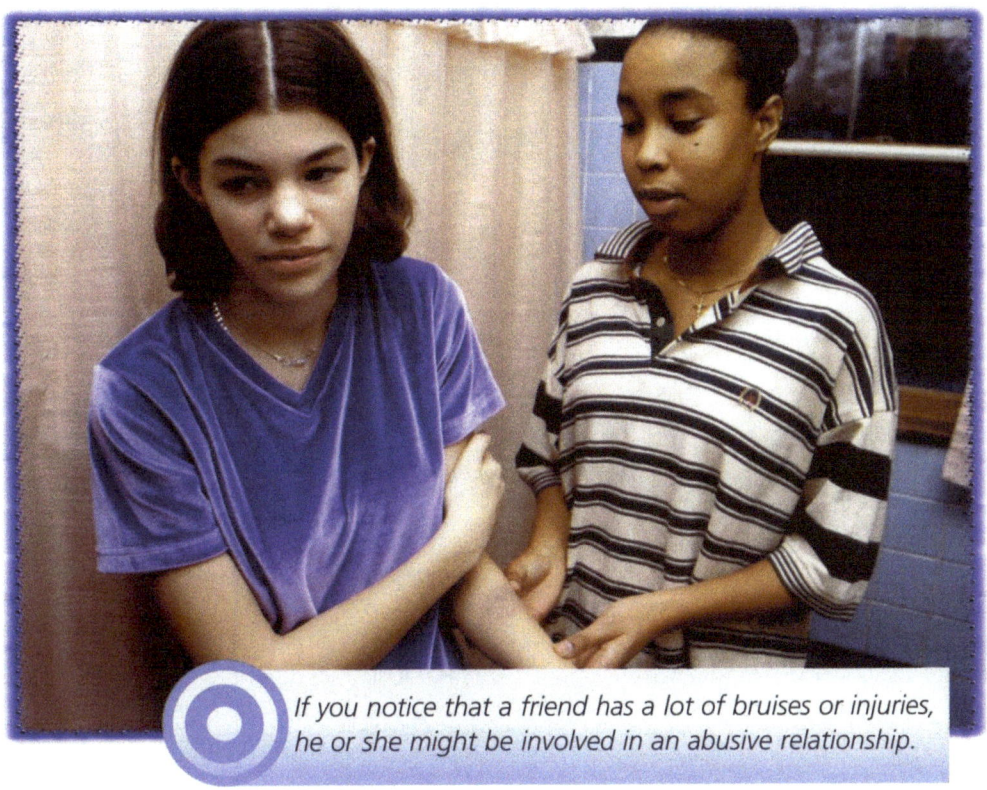

If you notice that a friend has a lot of bruises or injuries, he or she might be involved in an abusive relationship.

Confronting Your Friend

The most important thing you can do when you get together to talk with your friend is to be supportive. This means that attacking him or her for getting involved in this kind of situation will just not do. You need to approach this subject with extreme care and sensitivity. Imagine how hard this is on your friend. He or she may be scared for his or her life. Or he or she might not even know that what is happening to him or her is wrong.

Talk with your friend. Tell your friend what you have been seeing and ask how he or she feels about it. If your friend denies there is a problem, but you are

Relationship Violence

sure there is one, you may need to go to someone for help without your friend's permission. Although you might feel like a bad friend, in reality you are being the best one he or she could have. On the other hand, if your friend does open up and tells you that he or she is in an abusive relationship, stress to him or her how important it is to seek help.

Be sure to offer your support and guidance, but make clear that this situation is a serious one and an adult does need to be told. Perhaps if your friend does not want to tell someone alone, you can go with him or her. The best thing that you can do is offer your support and listen.

If You Are the Abuser

If you are the person who is doing the abusing in the relationship, by now you should know that you need to get some help. Your actions are not right, but there are things you can do to help yourself. Many of the sources listed in the back of this book can also be used by a person who has a tendency to be abusive, particularly Project PAVE. If you are not comfortable contacting this resource, then talk to someone you trust and maybe this person will help you find some resources.

Knowing that you have been abusive is a very hard thing to deal with. Many times, you have probably felt very out of control. But you can stop it. And now

Moving On

that you know you can, take the first step to change, and get help.

Combating Dating Violence

In an effort to combat the increase in dating violence, the news media has stepped up its coverage on the topic. Popular television is helping as well. In March 1999, *The Oprah Winfrey Show* dedicated an episode to women who abuse their husbands. These are just a few examples of what is being done to stop the rise of abusive and violent relationships.

Get Involved

Hopefully, after reading this book, you are aware that dating violence is not only a serious issue, but one that needs to be addressed. And you can be the person who makes the difference. You can begin by encouraging others to acknowledge the problem's existence and learn about what dating violence is and how it can be prevented. You can be proactive.

Increase Awareness

Making people aware of dating violence is one of the first steps toward reducing it. One way that you can do this is by putting up posters in your school and throughout your neighborhood that highlight the causes, warning signs, and, most important, the

Relationship Violence

resources that are available in your community that can offer help.

Another idea, from the Family Prevention Violence Fund, is to place safety cards in places that women frequent, like gyms, restaurants, or malls. These cards give details about domestic violence and dating violence that all men and women should know. They also allow people to pick them up anonymously, in case they are too embarrassed to tell someone that they are being abused.

If you are not ready to reach that far out into your community and interact with men and women of all ages, you can start by talking with your friends. Suggest books about the subject. Rent movies that you know will show them an abusive relationship. And make sure you tell each one of them why it is so important to stop the abuse as soon as it starts. Inform them that abuse is not just a one-time thing, even though their boyfriends or girlfriends will promise them that it was.

However, just as this book included information on healthy relationships, so should the knowledge and teachings that you share. It is just as vital that your friends know what makes a relationship good for them as it is that they be aware of what makes one bad. Their perspective, or ideas about relationships, should not be unbalanced. Instead, they need to be able to approach their relationships with some objectivity.

Moving On

In the Future

Dating violence is a subject that you will undoubtedly hear more and more about, and hopefully it will not be because of a violent incident like the Columbia University murder. Instead, as the media increases its coverage and various programs and Web sites like the ones listed in the Where to Go for Help section work toward awareness, knowledge will overcome, and the number of people who are involved in dating violence will decline.

Glossary

communication A key component of a healthy relationship, in which both partners exchange their ideas, perceptions, and beliefs.

compromise A settlement of a dispute in which the two sides each agree to accept less than they originally wanted.

dating violence A pattern of behavior in which a person tries to control his or her partner through psychological or physical acts of abuse.

emotional abuse Any behavior that is intended to cause psychological or emotional distress.

healthy relationship A relationship that has a mixture of communication, respect, trust, and compromise, and is void of abusive behavior.

Glossary

objectivity The ability to perceive or describe something without being influenced by personal emotions or prejudices.

physical abuse Any behavior that inflicts harm on a person's physical being.

respect To feel or show admiration toward somebody or something.

sexual abuse Any sexual behavior that makes a person feel uncomfortable, or sex that is forced.

trust To allow somebody to do or use something while having confidence that the person will behave responsibly or properly.

unhealthy relationship A type of relationship that is not based on trust, respect, communication, or compromise; instead, it tends to be abusive and destructive to one or both persons.

Where to Go for Help

In the United States

Advocates for Youth
1025 Vermont Avenue NW, Suite 200
Washington, DC 20005
(202) 347-5700
Web site: http://www.advocatesforyouth.org
e-mail: info@advocatesforyouth.org

The Alabama Coalition Against Domestic Violence
P.O. Box 4762
Montgomery, AL 36101
(334) 832-4842
Web site: http://www.acadv.org
e-mail: acadv@acadv.org

Where to Go for Help

Men Can Stop Rape
P.O. Box 57144
Washington, DC 20037-7144
(202) 265-6530
Web site: http://www.mencanstoprape.org
e-mail: info@mencanstoprape.org

National Crime Prevention Council
1000 Connecticut Avenue NW, 13th Floor
Washington, DC 20036
(202) 466-6272
Web site: http://www.ncpc.org

National Domestic Violence Hotline
(800) 799-SAFE (7233)

Project PAVE (Providing Alternatives to Violence)
2051 York Street
Denver, CO 80205
(303) 322-2382
e-mail: projectpave@uswest.net

SafeNetwork Project
Operated by the California District
 Attorneys Association
731 K Street, 3rd Floor
Sacramento, CA 95814

Relationship Violence

(916) 443-2017
Web site: http://www.safenetwork.net/teens/teens.html

A Window Between Worlds
710 4th Avenue, #4
Venice, CA 90291
(310) 396-0317
Web site: http://www.awbw.org
e-mail: window@awbw.org

In Canada

Canadian Research Institute for the Advancement of Women (CRIAW)
151 Slater Street, Suite 408
Ottawa, ON K1P 5H3
(613) 563-0681
Web site: http://www.criaw-icref.ca
e-mail: info@criaw-icref.ca

National Clearinghouse on Family Violence
Postal Locator 1907D1
Family Violence Prevention Division
Health Programs and Services Branch
Health Canada
Ottawa, ON K1A 1B4
(800) 267-1291 or (613) 957-2938

Where to Go for Help

Web site: http://www.hc-sc.gc.ca/
http/familyviolence/html/datingeng.html

Web Sites

Columbia/Barnard Rape Crisis/Anti-Violence
    Support Center
http://www.columbia.edu/cu/rcavsc/relationship.html

Cybergrrl.com
http://www.cybergrrl.com

DoSomething.org
http://www.dosomething.org

SafePlace Teensite
http://www.austin-safeplace.org/teens/index.htm

Violence Prevention Initiative
http://www.preventviolence.com

For Further Reading

Barbour, Scott. *Teen Violence.* San Diego, CA: Greenhaven Press, 1999.

Goldenstern, Joyce. *American Women Against Violence.* Springfield, NJ: Enslow Publishers, 1998.

Hicks, John. *Dating Violence: True Stories of Hurt and Hope.* Brookfield, CT: Millbrook Press, 1996.

Hipp, Earl. *Understanding the Human Volcano: What Teens Can Do About Violence.* Center City, MN: Hazeldon, 2000.

Levy, Barrie, ed. *Dating Violence: Young Women in Danger.* Seattle, WA: Seal Press, 1991.

Levy, Barrie. *In Love and in Danger: A Teen's Guide to Breaking Free of Abusive Relationships.* Seattle, WA: Seal Press, 1993.

For Further Reading

Lindquist, Scott. *The Date Rape Prevention Book: The Essential Guide for Girls and Women.* Naperville, IL: Sourcebooks, 2000.

Winkler, Kathleen. *Date Rape: A Hot Issue.* Springfield, NJ: Enslow Publishers, 1999.

Index

A
abuse, sexual, 14, 17, 18, 28
abuse, verbal/emotional, 13, 14, 15, 16–17, 18, 26, 28
abused friend, helping your, 47–50
abuser, if you are the, 50–51
abusive home, growing up in an, 19, 23–24
alcohol and drugs, 18, 24–26
anger, 24, 26
arguments, 8, 13, 21, 30, 48

B
behavior, healthy vs. unhealthy, 37

C
communication, 6, 31–32, 35, 37
compromise, 6, 33–34, 35
counselor/psychologist, 43–44, 45

F
friends, 16, 18, 21, 37, 40–41, 44, 47, 52–53

H
homosexual teens, 16

I
intuition/hunch, 42, 48

J
jealousy, 16, 18, 35

L
listening, 32–33
love, 6, 7, 36, 38

M
murder and suicide, 7, 18

P
parents, 7, 38, 40, 47
Project PAVE, 24, 50

R
relationships, abusive,
    getting out/leaving, 7, 8, 14, 18, 29, 35, 38, 39–42, 44

Index

recognizing, 7, 8, 19, 38, 39, 48
   telling adult about, 41
   telling someone about, 39–41, 44
relationships, healthy, 8, 24, 27–29, 30–35, 38, 52, 53
   bill of rights for, 34
relationship/dating violence
   excuses for, 36, 38
   it is never OK, 13, 14, 26, 27, 38
   men and women, 9, 26, 52
   myth that it happens only once, 13, 36, 52
   reasons why, 9, 19, 20–26
   in same-sex relationships, 16
   stopping it in your community, 38, 51–53
   what it is, 13
   who experiences it, 7, 20
relationship violence test, 18
respect, 30–31, 35, 37

S
safety cards, 52
safety guidelines, 44–47
self-respect/self-esteem, 15, 27, 43
stress, 20, 38

T
teen mothers, 27
trust, 15, 35, 50

V
violence around the world, 28
violence in the media, 19, 21

Y
yelling/screaming, 15, 32, 37

About the Author

Katherine White is a freelance writer who lives in Brooklyn, NY.

Photo Credits

Cover by Ira Fox; p. 2 by Cindy Reiman; p. 8 © Craig Witkowski/Index Stock; pp. 11, 12, 17, 22, 25, 28, 31, 33, 36, 41, 43, 46, 49 by Ira Fox.

Series Design

Tom Forget

Layout

Danielle Goldblatt

www.ingramcontent.com/pod-product-compliance
Lightning Source LLC
Chambersburg PA
CBHW041114070526
44584CB00002B/169